Junk Food: The Answer Book

Books in This Series

Fitness: The Answer Book by Cecil B. Murphey

Flab: The Answer Book by Jim Krafft, M.D.

Headaches: The Answer Book by Joan Miller, Ph.D.

Heart Attacks: The Answer Book by Daniel J. MacNeil, M.D., and Larry Losoncy, Ph.D.

Junk Food: The Answer Book by Virginia and Norman Rohrer

Vitamins: The Answer Book by Virginia and Norman Rohrer

JUNK FOOD
The Answer Book

Virginia and Norman Rohrer

SPIRE BOOKS

Fleming H. Revell Company
Old Tappan, New Jersey

ISBN: 0-8007-8467-7

A Spire Book

Printed in the United States of America

CONTENTS

INTRODUCTION

"Junk food" is a coined phrase that quite accurately describes food with excessive sugar, fat, salt, and preservatives, which millions of Americans put into their stomachs every day. Physicians see the harmful effects of modern diet perhaps more than anyone else.

I heartily endorse any appeal that warns against the indulgence of poor eating and drinking habits, but I am especially enthusiastic about the message of this book because I know the authors and their life-styles. If more people practiced what this book preaches, we physicians might be out of jobs! Certainly there would be healthier babies, brighter youngsters, fewer teenagers in trouble with the law, less depression among adults, fewer divorces, and longer life.

What better reason does anyone need for eating right and feeling great?

We would all be beneficiaries if our refrigerators never saw the sodium nitrites and nitrates of cured meats (frankfurters, bologna, salami, corned beef, bacon, and ham). These preservatives have actually been shown to cause cancer in laboratory animals, yet the government still allows us to place into our shopping carts large selections of these chemically laced foods.

This book is delightfully informative and motivating. You're going to like it! You're also going to like the English French toast (page 54)—a delectable treat even without the usual sop of syrup that has become for most of us a lifelong reflex.

ROBERT G. WELLS, M.D.

PREFACE

Ever since food processors began to denature food and substitute chemicals for nutrients, junk food has been a part of the "civilized" diet. This greasy, breaded, fried, salty, spicy, heavily sweetened, chemically treated, and additive-laden food is characteristic of the fast-food phenomenon in America today. The industry dangles temptingly before our appetites hot dogs, French fries, doughnuts, frozen desserts, thick shakes, and soft drinks as children grow fat, teeth decay, resilience softens, and muscles grow flabby.

Junk food was introduced in the 1940s when mom needed something quick in order to get back to the factory during World War II, while her soldier husband on the front lines was eating Spam and other artificial rations. In the 1950s junk food flourished, as hamburgers, fried chicken, and other specialties in quick-service restaurants and take-out shops became popular.

Convenience foods were heralded as a major step forward. With less time needed for simmering and basting, the frozen foods in disposable tins seemed like blessings. Children's lunches were also easier. Thanks to modern food technology, mom no longer needed to braise the brisket for sandwiches. She simply popped in those prepackaged chips. Soon youngsters discovered the delights of putting luncheon meats between white bread and munching the soft dough. The brown bread was for peasants or those strange vegetarians down the street who didn't know any better or who were so lacking in culture that they had not taken the step toward refinement.

Twinkies, Oreo cookies, and other such tasties became

available when commerce and science joined forces to distribute the nation's food. At the same time, Americans were moving from farms to cities, and family life in the United States was undergoing drastic changes. The automobile gave young people mobility, and convenience foods went hand-in-hand with the revolution.

In the sixties, waves of young Americans "dropped out" of American society to create a kind of counterculture. They expressed their dissatisfaction with what President Eisenhower had called the military-industrial complex, let their hair grow long, and put big-business food chains on their "hit list." They formed rural communes and began to grow and raise their own food "naturally" or "organically," that is, without the use of synthetic fertilizers, pesticides, fungicides, or growth hormones. Others became vegetarians and devotees of raw foods, or of yogurt and honey, wheat germ, and alfalfa sprouts with natural vitamin therapy. American society tolerantly dubbed this group "the granola generation."

Big business, ever watchful of the market, jumped on the bandwagon. Next to the sugar-coated corn, rice, and other refined cereals stood boxes of products labeled "everything natural, nothing artificial."

Still, the phenomenon of the fat teenager is a serious problem in America today. How can we lure young people away from the empty calories, grease, salt, and sugar that play havoc with body and soul? Remember: Love is not equal to the amount of food your child eats. Love sometimes grows more with less.

Let's make a start.

Junk Food: The Answer Book

Inside his grass house Courtney stirred his steaming pots and sang his morning song:

Blackstrap molasses
Wheat germ bread
Live so long
Wish you were dead

"Watcha makin' this time?" asked Tiny Mo as he rode up on his bike.

"I'm making my Chewsday dish," Courtney called through the window. "Want some?"

"Naw, I'm eating chocolate pie from Mr. Johnson's market."

"That's not chocolate pie," Courtney corrected.

"It's not?" Tiny Mo asked, looking at the wrapper.

Courtney wiped his hands on his apron and went outside. "See this label?" he asked. "You are eating diglycerides, cellulose gum, polysorbate 80, carrageenan, sodium caseinate, artificial color, and yellow dye five. It's a wonder you don't have a stomachache."

"I do, sometimes," Tiny Mo said.

"And are you tired in the afternoon?" asked Courtney.

"Yes. I can't sit still in school, can't sleep very well at night, and I already have holes in my teeth."

"Well, then," said Courtney, "you better come inside and eat some real food with me. I've got wake-up-feeling-fine food, energy-in-the-afternoon food, sit-still-in-school food, teeth-without-holes food, and go-to-sleep-at-night food."

"Hurrah!" said Tiny Mo.

1

The Mad Chemists

No one in that dreadful winter of 1609 in the Virginia Colony spoke of "junk food" or "health food." They spoke rather of possible starvation.

No pioneer breaking virgin soil in Kentucky in 1790 even dreamed of "instant" foods prepared in a minute by adding water or heating.

No sodbuster on the Great Plains in 1880 ever gave any thought to whether or not his crops were organically produced, although of course they were.

Until 1897, all the food—vittles, chow, grub, mess, or chuck—that Americans ate was naturally grown and processed. Jerky, strips of smoked or sun-dried venison or other game meat, was a gift from the Indians. The German (Pennsylvania Dutch) settlers learned how to dry apples for their schnitz. New Englanders "corned" their beef, and Southerners smoke-cured hams, bacon, and other hog-butchered cuts. Some vegetables were preserved by pickling; cabbage became sauerkraut; root cellars held vege-

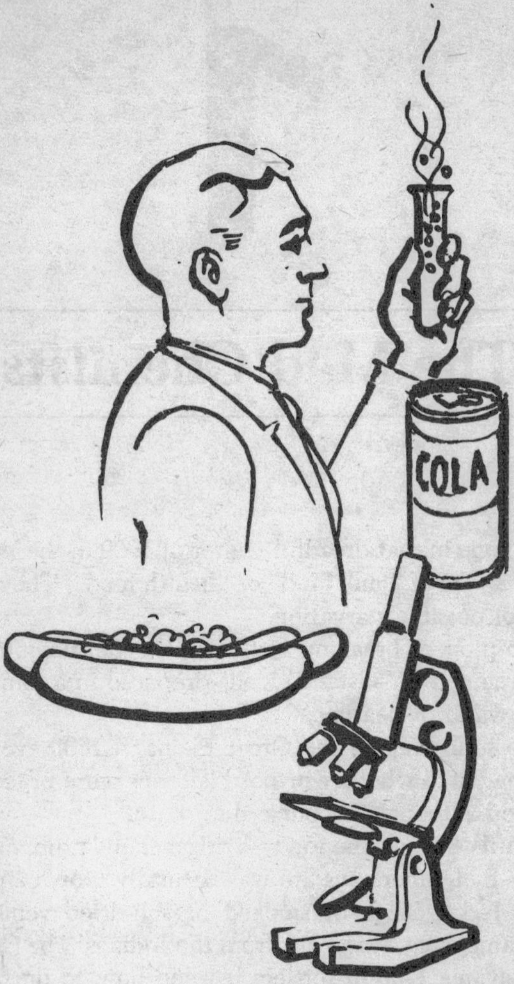

The twentieth century has brought us food products developed in chemical laboratories.

tables like potatoes, onions, beets, carrots, turnips, parsnips, and rutabagas all winter.

A heat-sealing process for canning that killed bacteria was introduced in the early 1800s by a Frenchman named Nicolas Appert to provide healthful foods for Napoleon's soldiers. The Civil War in the United States (1861–65) hastened the production of foods in tin cans such as tomatoes, pork and beans, sauerkraut, and fruit.

Canned evaporated milk appeared in the mid-1800s and was popularized by Gail Borden, a man whose name was used by a large dairy. City dwellers without cows could now enjoy milk that was safe and tasty. Pasteurization (heating fresh milk to kill harmful bacteria) was introduced in the late 1890s.

Railroad refrigerator cars and the household icebox (forerunner of the modern automatic electric refrigerator) revolutionized the food-processing and distribution industries of the country.

In 1897 scientists in a lab produced a shimmering, colorful gelatin-based mass that soon found a place on every American shelf and was considered to be wholesome and healthful—the perfect dessert for children, dieters, invalids—everybody! Actually, such desserts are less than nutritionally adequate. High in refined sugar and synthetic additives, they tend to contain only 10 percent gelatin, which offers a poor quality protein at best.

Americans eagerly bought the tinted-sugar formula in the early 1900s. Coal-tar-dye-colored, imitation-fruit-flavored commodities, powdered and liquid soft drinks and confections quickly followed the new dessert into the stomachs of the brave sons of the New World.

The process of freezing food was introduced by Brooklyn-born inventor Clarence Birdseye. He noticed during a trip to Labrador in the early 1900s that fish drawn from the sea in subfreezing temperatures and quickly frozen by nature tasted as delicious as fresh fish when thawed and cooked. Flash freezing mechanically, he discovered, kept the tissues of meat and vegetables from breaking down. He patented the process in 1920 and launched the modern frozen-food industry.

Canning, refrigeration, freezing—all splendid advances for the food industry—led naturally to synthetic and artificial substitutes for nature's best. In 1897 the chemists might have put on the label, "everything artificial, nothing natural," and Americans would have applauded the catch line. But we've had the piper to pay for our sins.

There is, however, the rumbling of drumbeats across the land. The call back to "live" foods and national health has begun. An apron is the banner of this marching army, kitchen cutlery, its weapons as the army of ex-junkies marches against bankrupt foods that are weakening and killing this generation.

Join the revolution! The results of yesterday's bad habits can't be totally remedied, but all who are willing to change should be prepared for some happy surprises.

2

How Kids Get Trapped

In the daytime I'm Mister Natural,
Just as healthy as I can be.
But at night I'm a Junk Food Junkie,
Good Lord, have pity on me.

Thus crooned Larry Groce in 1974. Children snickered, parents smiled. Each went on eating 125 to 130 pounds of refined sugar every year, 55 pounds of fat, 300 cans or bottles of soda pop, 200 sticks of chewing gum, more than 20 gallons of ice cream, 18 pounds of candy, 5 pounds of potato chips, a couple more pounds of pretzels and corn chips, 63 dozen doughnuts, and some 50 pounds of cookies and cakes—each loving every empty calorie, tempting malnutrition, reducing energy levels, and inviting the syndrome of low blood sugar (hypoglycemia) and diabetes.

Taste Buds Rule the Head

Why do junkies enjoy their addiction and make no effort to break their habit even when told of the dangers? From birth, we learn to prefer foods that taste sweet. The first nourishment that passes through our mouths is milk—mother's or cow's—which contains lactose, one of nature's basic sugars.

"The primary function of taste sensitivity [is to] determine which parts of the environment contain substances suitable as food and which do not," explains Dr. R. J. Watson of the Department of Nutrition at the University of London. "Of the four basic taste sensations—sweet, salty, sour, bitter—the first two [are associated] with the possible presence of food and the last two indicate the use of possible harmful substances."

Flavor, say the behavioral psychologists, is probably the most important characteristic in satisfying the instinctive craving that is common to all. Experience determines which flavors are acceptable. The palate does not necessarily select those foods that make up a well-balanced, nutritious diet. The brainwashing of advertising lures us into the sweetened, oily, and salted fare whose flavors dance delightfully on the tongue.

Children are taught to look upon sweets as rewards. No clean plate—no dessert is the common admonition. So dinner is endured and dessert becomes a reward.

Hidden sugars in presweetened breakfast cereals with up to 68 percent refined sugar are the most successful in fostering the junk-food habit.

"Refined sugar is an incomplete food," says William Dufty, author of *Sugar Blues.* "All nutrients have been processed out. Incomplete foods are addicting. If a body is nourished, it has a cutoff point for foods it has obtained enough of, a natural reaction. But with incomplete foods such as refined sugar, the body is fooled and continually demands more and more. It can't get its fill."

Literature supports the contention that anything sweet is good. Shakespeare writes in *Hamlet*, "Sweets to the sweet, farewell!" Samson, in the Old Testament of the Bible, proclaims, "Out of the eater came forth meat, and out of the strong came forth sweetness." Parents say, "Be nice to your sister; you'll get more with honey than with vinegar."

Western civilization gets the message and gags on it. Radio and TV ads bombard our ears, and our heart responds to the tongue's demands. Impressionable, growing children sink deeper and deeper into the morass.

3

Adding Up the Additives

Junk-food catchwords include *additive, artificial,* and *chemical.* Americans once welcomed such laboratory discoveries as saccharin and heralded them as beneficial. Today they are seen as detrimental because time has uncovered the dangers to the human body of a number of synthetic substances added to food.

The highly toxic dyes developed in the mid-1800s gave luster to the new civilized foods. Brightly colored candies appealed to the eye, as well as the taste, of children. Federal food laws were passed in 1906 because of spoiled beef sold during the Spanish-American War. This situation uncovered scandalous conditions in the meat-packing plants. Other harmful, impure, and polluted food products surfaced until the sweeping Food, Drug, and Cosmetic Act was passed in 1938 to fight such outrages as "raspberry jam" consisting of gelatinous sugar mixtures with hayseeds!

The shelves of a supermarket today offer some 3,000 additives. Their strengths, hazards, and potential damage cause widespread confusion not only for the consumer but also for the Food and Drug Administration. The FDA can authorize or prohibit the use of an additive. The chemicals and preservatives added *since* 1958 (when the Food Additives Amendment was passed by Congress) are assumed to be safe after adequate testing by their sponsors. Those on the market *before* 1958 were not pretested. These were lumped by the FDA into a middle category commonly called GRAS (generally recognized as safe) to await testing at a later date. Of the approximately 600 or so pre-1958 additives, only about half have been reviewed so far. Most have been stamped "safe," but not all.

Long-term effects and the interaction of additives with other chemicals make the testing process tedious. Laboratory experiments cannot tell the full story. To be safe, more and more people are avoiding additive-laden foods—even the ones branded "safe."

Artificial Versus Natural

Is a natural substance from plants more safe than the chemical combinations from a laboratory? Is molasses extract from sugar used for coloring safe? How about gelatin from bones used for thickening? They're natural, so why aren't they totally safe?

The answer is: because all natural substances aren't totally safe. Caffeine and quinine are good examples of natural substances that can harm the body. Caffeine destroys vitamin B_1 and makes the body jittery. Coffee consumption is now implicated in cancer of the bladder. The gum tragacanth taken from plants and used as a stabilizer in salad dressings can cause swelling of tissues and breathing difficulty in the allergic individual. So can excessive use of sugar, mustard, and pepper along with many other spices, herbs, and extracts.

Keep in mind that numerous additives taken from natural sources, such as vegetable gums, milk casein, and hydrolyzed vegetables are doctored with laboratory compounds in the process of manufacturing them. The consumer cannot always separate the natural from the artificial and cannot always label one good and the other bad. *Natural* bacteria, yeasts, and fungi can poison and kill. Sodium benzoate, on the other hand, is a laboratory chemical that can retard food spoilage and prevent illness and death.

Few Americans can dine on fresh foods daily, so additives will be part of our food supply for a long time. It's a trade off. But it's still wise to bake and freeze your own bread to avoid benzoated sodas as much as possible. It's still wise to avoid sodium *nitrate* and sodium *nitrite* in cured meats and fish (frankfurters, bologna, salami, corned beef, bacon, and ham). These chemicals retard spoilage and stop the growth of deadly botulism bacteria. They also give these foods the red coloring and flavor to which our taste has become accustomed. However, in the stomach, nitrates and nitrites are converted into nitrosamines, which have caused cancer in laboratory animals. Bacon is a high-risk food because the high-heat cooking period results in increased bodily concentration of nitrosamines. To all this is added the high salt content of cured meats, making them items to leave off the shopping list.

Synthetic additives do more than prevent spoilage. They add color, flavor, leavening agents (baking soda, baking powder), and bleaching agents (for whitened flour) and thicken, stabilize, emulsify, and tantalize the hungry eye.

Purists tend to reject foods fortified artificially with the B vitamins, iron, calcium, and vitamins A and D, which are added commercially to many cereals and dairy products.

Unfortunately, manufacturers advertise products "fortified" with synthetic vitamins and minerals as "abundantly nutritious" because they are "enriched." The consumer would be far ahead to gain these nutrients in pure fruit juices, whole grains, and fresh fruits rather than in the food to which they have been artificially added in smaller amounts.

Cheap ingredients such as gums and emulsifiers that artificially color or flavor or make creamy are additional dangers because they can be substituted for egg whites or cream and thus result in a bigger profit while shortchanging the customer nutritionally and economically.

The culprits Red Dye No. 2 and Red Dye No. 4 have been stricken from the safe list, but others are still being served that are potentially dangerous. One is Red Dye No. 40, which is carcinogenic in animals, and another is Yellow Dye No. 5, which is allergenic to humans. Food processors do not always comply with orders to eliminate banned dyes and often continue to use them to our detriment. It's best, therefore, to avoid all foods containing artificial coloring as much as possible.

Astutely avoid also such additives as BHT (butylated hydroxytoluene). These antioxidants are added to prevent rancidity in fat-containing products like potato chips, corn chips, and salad oils. They serve also to maintain freshness and extend shelf life in dry cereals, cake mixes, chewing gums, and candies.

Yet another culprit among additives is BVO (brominated vegetable oil). This emulsifier is put into citrus-flavored soft drinks to disperse the cloudy citrus portion throughout the beverage. Its residue is poisonous and can be stored in body tissues.

An additive that is difficult to avoid is MSG (monosodium glutamate), an effective flavor enhancer occurring naturally in seaweed, soybeans, and sugar beets. Asians have used it for years, but it has only been used commercially in the United States since the early 1900s. MSG spices up the flavor of factory-prepared soups, sauces, stews, and seasoning mixtures. It makes meat and poultry dishes taste more "beefy" or "chickeny" than they really are. Chinese food often contains heavy doses. MSG can cause dizziness and/or headaches. Some people suffer a numbness in the head, neck, chest, and arms after ingesting it.

Adults can tolerate MSG better than children, throwing off the aftereffects in about an hour or two. However, the public cried out angrily when tests showed that MSG damaged brain cells in baby mice. It was banned from baby foods, but MSG is still on the GRAS list for many foods that young children eat. Some foods like mayonnaise and salad dressings contain MSG without the requirement that it be named on the ingredients label.

Additives in Whole Food

Restaurant fare and processed foods carry the most additives, but growers, raisers, packers, and distributors have so tampered with edibles that even whole food is tainted by additives.

DDT, in the 1940s, was hailed as the miracle substance that would save vast amounts of crops from destruction by hungry insects. But by the time the testing laboratories caught up with the hazards, residues of DDT had built up in soil, water, plants, animals, and humans. Chemicals called PCBs (polychlorinated biphenyls) have also invaded, leaving minute toxic deposits in plant life, sea life, and in the tissues of animal and human body fat.

Add to these the dozens of pesticides, fungicides, herbicides, and synthetic fertilizers, and the contaminants become even more widespread. Some ranchers medicate their poultry and cattle with tranquilizers and antibiotics for maximum weight at the marketplace, but those chemicals tend to concentrate in the fatty tissues and livers of the animals that eat them. Then they are passed on in cumulative amounts to meat-eating humans.

There are more contaminants in our "silent spring": gases, dyes, and waxes used on fruits and vegetables to make them more attractive to the consumer who likes food that is glossy and vividly colored (just as in the magazine and TV ads). Tomatoes picked green far away and reddened en route to market by ethylene gas have fewer vitamins. Green oranges are colored artificially with Citrus Red No. 2 (suspected of being carcinogenic). The dye doesn't leak into the pulp, but some manufacturers use that same dye-soaked rind in marmalade, baking, or other cooking, and that's what is harmful. Industry caucuses rose up and successfully demanded an end to the "color added" label on the rind.

Labels With Missing Ingredients

Whole foods should contain information about the dyes, waxes, gases, and other spoilage retardants and cosmetic enhancers added, but most often they do not. The FDA reasons that these conform to its "standard of identity" for that product. That means, if a jar of mayonnaise contains a certain amount of vegetable oil, plus lemon juice or vinegar, and egg yolks, it can be labeled simply "mayonnaise" (although MSG is probably among its flavor enhancers with salt, sugar, and spices).

When manufacturers began substituting more and more additives and fake ingredients, a movement was started to take some processed foods out of the "assumed" category. Ice cream is an example. This cool smoothy lost its "standard of identity" status in July 1979. Thereafter, manufacturers were required to list all ingredients on the label (except artificial coloring). The powerful dairy industry forced the government to back off on requirements concerning artificial coloring.

A Discouraging Word

The overall picture of contaminated food intake in America can be discouraging: Coke-guzzling children wandering on caffeine highs; adults with headaches from Chinese restaurant syndrome (MSG); breakfast bacon with cancer-causing preservatives sizzling in the pan; potato chips loaded with BHT; soda pop with BVO; orange skins dyed with dangerous artificial coloring; once-edible apples coated with wax—all this while the cumbersome governmental regulatory red tape, the testing inadequacies, and the threat of business loss threatens to make improvement slowly, if ever, realized.

The Escape

Try to avoid as much additive-laden processed foods as possible. Whole foods are best. Seek food that has traveled the shortest distance from farm to market with the fewest intermediate agents. Eat in-season fruits and vegetables from farm stands and products from local egg and dairy farms.

When supermarket fruits and vegetables are bought, scrub edible skins with a brush and a nontoxic liquid cleanser. No residue will be left as might be the case when using a detergent. Leafy vegetables can be rinsed in salt water for cleansing and to float out the tiny bugs from down in the leaves.

Eat in fast-food restaurants less frequently. Resist the

temptation to consume junk "just this once." It's always harder to resist the next time.

Failure to take action, as the next chapter warns, could be regrettable.

4

The Media Blitz

Ever since 1868 when George Mortimer Pullman designed a dining car for speeding trains, Americans have been eating on the go. Kids today are eating not only on the go but also on the run.

Michael S. Lasky, in his book *The Complete Junk Food Book*, refers to junk food made and sold expressly for children as "kiddie litter." The manufacturers of sodas, cereals, and candy blanket schoolyards with free literature, which nutritionists brand as downright lies.

One of these booklets distributed by the National Confectioners' Association to some 60,000 students and teachers makes the following claims:

- Candy is vital for weight watchers. "To reduce, eat candy before and/or after each meal. We can promise you it works!"
- Candy plays a decisive role as a fever fighter and actually prevents vomiting, diarrhea, and convulsions.
- Cavities in your teeth are caused by "the lack of use of

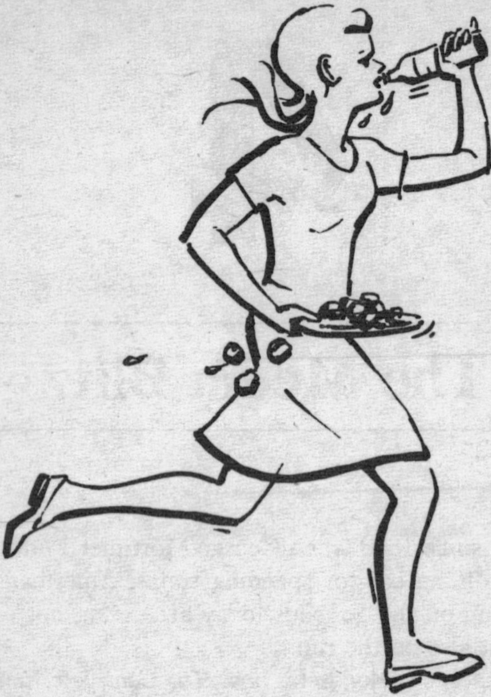

Many of our "meals" are snacks eaten on the run.

the teeth in hard chewing." Candy is passed off as only a minor source of dental decay.

The National Soft Drink Association tells youngsters that soda is "a good source of water." In that case, replies Dr. Michael Jacobson, codirector of the Center for Science in the Public Interest, "it would be better to drink water."

Dr. Jean Mayer, popular columnist on nutrition for major newspapers across the nation, maintains that the literature on "kiddie litter" is "outrageous, misleading, and contrary to fact."

General Foods, manufacturers of Post cereals, once launched a multimillion-dollar advertising program in which the company offered to donate gym equipment to schools that collected specified numbers of Post cereal box tops. Their letters lamented that in the current money crunch much-needed physical education equipment could not be obtained by cost-cutting school boards. Here was a free way to get it. The school principals were put in the position of having to endorse certain cereals to get the box tops in order to get the gym equipment, and many did so enthusiastically.

TV Lure

Television is still the direct line to a child's imagination. The "box" lures them relentlessly to partake of sugary sweet foods. The Broadcast Advertisers Report says that the young TV viewer is hit an average of twenty times an hour with invitations to enjoy some sugary sweet food. This compares to seven to nine commercials an hour on prime-time adult programming. Each commercial is targeted toward the impressionable child.

Robert B. Choate, a critic of TV ads for youngsters, told the Senate Subcommittee on the Consumer (which was investigating TV advertising to children): "When you take a child who sits and watches television from the age of two to ten or eleven and sits in front of the Saturday morning TV box and listens to sugar, sugar, sugar, sweetness, sweetness, sweetness, chocolate, chocolate, chocolate, that child picks up a habit which is going to continue through life."

A contingent of outraged teachers and parents formed the Action for Children's Television in the early 1970s and formally complained to the Federal Communications Commission and the Federal Trade Commission. In one of

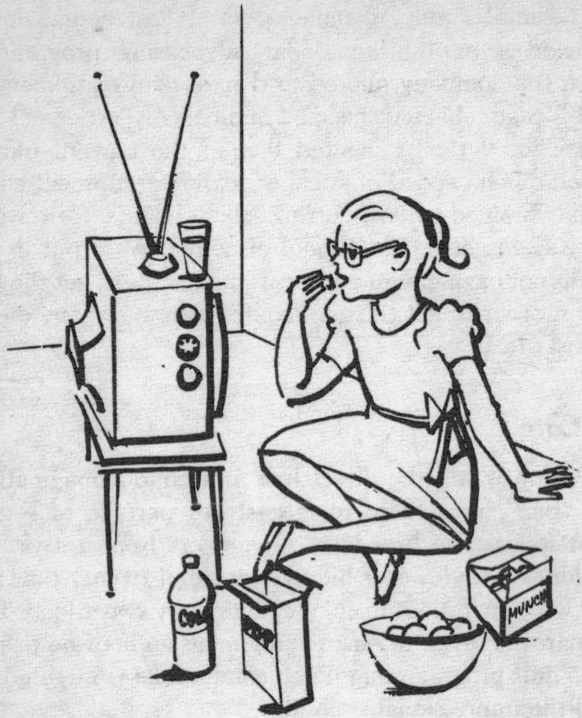

Television commercials have a strong impact on children's food choices.

their petitions to the FTC, Action for Children's Television (ACT) documented the misinformation and false ideals that kiddie-litter commercials provided for American youngsters.

A chief complaint of ACT was that parental advice was pitted against TV ads that "come fast and furious." The group noted that cereal, one of the hallowed "basics"—a food TV tells them is part of a balanced diet—is advertised only on the merits of being "super sweet." The youngsters are taught to equate eating the "goodies" with basic human values.

Michael Lasky notes the appeal of the ads in this outline:

> BROTHERHOOD: "Learn brotherhood," croons Post's Sugar Bear, "and we *all* love Super Sugar Crisp. Share it with your friends."
>
> FRIENDSHIP: Joe Namath introduces a young boy to his "old pals"—various football stars—and finally to his *old pal,* Ovaltine.
>
> POWER: "Have breakfast with the King." King Vitaman Cereal.
>
> COMMON SENSE: "If you put Sweet Pebble in your mouth, you'll never have rocks in your head."
>
> HAPPINESS: "There's nothing like the face of a kid eating a Hershey bar, there's nothing like it you'll ever see, a face as happy as it can be."
>
> FUN: "You get a big delight in every bite." Hostess Cupcakes.
>
> ECOLOGY: "Help, Blob is polluting the ocean." But Sugar Bear in his best Bing Crosby voice comes to the rescue bearing Super Sugar Crisp and triumphing over evil.

The Surgeon General's Scientific Advisory Committee on TV and Social Behavior studied children subjected to television's barrage. It found that the junk-food products advertised on TV are more frequently requested by the child than other products.

The Cereal Institute, a public-relations wing of the cereal-processing industry, estimated that 1 billion "backsides" are shown to Americans each year—that's like half a million billboards by space. Most of the backs of packages carry hype on toy premiums or free items that are sent in exchange for boxtops.

(Note: Four of the major cereal manufacturers now own toy companies.)

While thousands of people are dying every day from

starvation, our children in America consume millions of pounds of food that is not nourishing their bodies but merely filling up the hunger space. There is cause for lamentation on both counts.

5

Delinquency and Junk Food

A thin, sullen teenager stepped up to the window of a quick-order restaurant in Los Angeles and asked for "the usual" lunch—a Coke and large fries.

The clock stood at 12:15 P.M. In forty-five minutes he faced an examination in French. After that, algebra and gym classes before school would be dismissed for another day.

The teenager bolted his junk food and sped back to campus in his hopped-up Chevy, "fortified" with a lunch that had given him a mountain of sugar, a shot of caffeine, with a dash of fat and salt. At breakfast that morning he had had a doughnut and a cup of coffee.

That evening at home the boy was irritable and jumpy. Too tired to do his homework and too nervous to eat a full dinner, he reacted angrily to each suggestion that he eat. He argued with his parents at every opportunity, finally hurling at them a barrage of verbal abuse as he stormed out of the house and sped away in his car. At a little past midnight his parents were notified that their son had taken the police on a high-speed chase. The boy had failed to make a turn in the road and hit a concrete retaining wall. He suffered severe lacerations as he was thrown out of the hurtling car.

Could diet explain the teenager's erratic behavior?

In high school, Skip Hanson of Cleveland was friendly and alert, competitive in sports, and well liked on campus. The future looked bright for this youthful entrepreneur as he made the principal's honor roll. Skip won a place on the All-League First Team basketball squad and looked the picture of health.

"On the exterior," Skip said, "I was aggressive and high strung. In reality, I suffered from painful depression."

After high school Skip accepted a scholarship to play basketball at Northwestern University, alternating between hyperactivity and extreme fatigue, which always preceded depression. He tried desperately to put aside his emotions and continued to play basketball, rising to the position of second leading scorer and rebounder.

"Peer pressure and the teaching of a great coach drove me on," Skip recalls. "But I began slowly to lose my battle. I felt like quitting everything, but I was unable to say no to the increasing demands of the game."

Several physicians and psychologists offered their explanations of Skip's wide mood swings. Finally he lost his grip. He turned down the scholarship and withdrew into himself.

One afternoon he could stand the pain no longer. He swallowed forty-eight sleeping pills, locked himself in his parents' garage, and started the car engine, prepared to die.

An alert mail carrier strolled by, heard the motor running inside the garage and called the paramedics. The quick work of the professionals saved Skip's life. Megavitamin therapy gave dramatic relief for what was later diagnosed as a biochemical and metabolic upset. He had pushed his body too long without an adequate and nutritious diet. There was not adequate fuel for his demanding schedule.

On a trip to a convention in Chicago, we found ourselves circling O'Hare airport for forty-five minutes, waiting for our turn to land.

"May I sit here?" asked a teenager as she popped into a seat on the aisle.

"Of course," we replied to this scraggly girl with worn-out jeans, soiled blouse, and sloppy grooming.

"I need a cigarette, and I can't smoke up there."

We had boarded late and found seats only in the foul air of the smoking section.

In the conversation that followed during the holding pattern aloft we learned that eighteen-year-old Rhonda had been released from jail the day before and was flying to Philadelphia to be with her mother and stepfather.

"What was your diet like in prison?" we asked.

"Well, for breakfast we had strong coffee, doughnuts, and other bakery stuff," Rhonda replied.

"How about lunch?"

"Well, that was canned peaches, spaghetti, white bread, and coffee. Supper maybe a sandwich, salt, two cookies, and more coffee."

She acted surprised when we urged her to eat more nutritious food now that she was out of jail. Before running away, Rhonda had paid little attention to what she ate. Food was food—and the more sugary, salty, breaded, fatty, and fluffy the better.

Was junk food the reason she could not get along with her parents? Could a lack of vitamins and minerals be the cause of her trembling hand, her fear of meeting her loved ones at the end of her trip? What about the lines of fatigue, pallor, and pimples that marred the face of this winsome, spindly youngster? Would she continue to drink coffee, Coke, and other soda pop, to smoke, and to punish her youthful body even in the freedom beyond the prison bars?

Charlie Brown, in the Peanuts comic strip, once asked his "psychiatrist" (Lucy in her booth) what caused his depression. He poured out an anguished appeal for help, listing his woes, his fears, and his feelings of despair.

Lucy stuck out her palm and said, "Your blood sugar is low. Five cents, please."

The diagnosis might have helped Charlie Brown's tensions for a brief period, but eventually they would return unless he did something about that biochemical upset.

"All emotions have biochemical as well as psychological elements," according to Abraham Hoffer, M.D., director of psychiatric research in Saskatchewan's Department of Public Health.

Dr. Richard Horace Hoffmann believes that "most neurotics are the way they are because some underlying and undiscovered bodily ailment contributes to their anxiety."

For a nickel, Charlie Brown had discovered a clue to his ailment—that the metabolism of the body directly affects the emotions. Until Charlie tunes up his anatomy, no amount of psychological counseling will totally eliminate his agonies.

It cost Terry more than a nickel to find out the cause of his ailments. Terry was a jittery, twenty-four-year-old man who was locked into a pattern of seeing a psychologist because "something terrible was wrong." He was afraid of crowds, afraid of becoming a captive, afraid to wander very far from home, afraid of a rapid pulse, and afraid of fear itself.

Doctors had prescribed hypnotherapy, psychotherapy, acupuncture, and behavioral therapy. His general health was good, but depression was worse than poor health, he concluded.

A friend directed Terry to a doctor who tested him for hypoglycemia. A six-hour glucose-tolerance examination showed the typical saw-tooth curve—two distinct peaks—with the chart showing definite drops of the blood-sugar level to dangerous readings.

He was given a carefully prescribed diet, but he found splendid and wonderful reasons for not keeping to it. After that first visit he went on a trip and then returned for another session with the doctor. This time he kept to his diet. His report:

"I'm sleeping better, have more sex drive, don't have constipation, and generally feel more confident."

After eating less refined sugars and carbohydrates, he reported that lingering headaches and pain in the right upper back was letting go. He felt like a new man.

The whole thrust of junk food and behavior was the focus of the First Annual Convention of the Feingold Association of the United States held in Washington, D.C. The sponsor was Dr. Benjamin F. Feingold, a physician long associated with the Kaiser-Permanente Health Care Program in San Francisco.

The diet that Dr. Feingold sets forth for children who are hyperkinetic eliminates all foods containing artificial coloring or flavoring, and all salicylates (substances found in artificial form in most headache pills and in natural form in certain fruits and vegetables—chiefly apples, peaches, oranges, cucumbers, and tomatoes).

Each parent at the Feingold convention had experienced heartbreaking episodes with their out-of-control children. Each, after a change of diet for the child, had seen dramatic changes for the better. Some referred to the change as a miracle.

The New York State United Teachers Association, with 2,000 delegates present, passed a resolution accepting Dr. Feingold's theory on food additives and the bad effect additives have on the hyperactive children. They even went on record opposing food additives for children *and* teachers!

One elementary school has instructed teachers to show children how to read labels. Anything with the word *artificial* cannot be brought into classrooms of that school.

A dietitian in another school ordered the kitchen to bake all the breads, cakes, and cookies it served. The official gave the order to serve only white cheeses with no colorings or additives. Chocolate milk and soft drinks were banned.

The national Feingold organization seeks to persuade food manufacturers to provide more complete and detailed labeling on products for sale. One processor correctly labeled his food "pure," but children were still reacting after ingesting it. The reason was quickly discovered: The package in which the food was sold had been treated with chemicals. These were absorbed into the food and set hyperkinetic children on a tirade.

The University of California at Los Angeles, with its vast biomedical research facilities, has taken an interest in children and their diets. In a "Child Study Program" UCLA studied hyperactive boys aged nine to twelve who are now receiving methylphenidate (Ritalin) medication to keep them emotionally and physically stable. Harvard and Yale Universities, smaller colleges, and increasing numbers of medical facilities are budgeting for research in this vital area, as more and more ex-junkies want to kick the habit and make their bodies (and emotions) stronger.

"We can do without food colorings," says the Psycho-Pharmacological Bulletin of April 1978, "but we can't do away with additives."

The elimination of additives used as preservatives would indeed limit our choices of food. But what is more important: our national health or tickling our taste buds? The motive, in the last analysis, is commercial profit.

Problem children in America often are suffering from the malnutrition of affluence, which manifests itself as psychoses. Because of the heavy onslaught of refined grain and sugar, an unstable blood sugar is often a result and a cause of emotional instability.

Doctors Gilles Lortie and Dean M. Laird, psychiatrists at the Worcester State Hospital in Massachusetts, have noted that such emotional instability includes the "inability to speak properly, purposeless movements, incoordination, silliness, negativism, twitching, incoherence, and mental dullness."

The physicians noted also that these symptoms have at times been improperly diagnosed as epilepsy, alcoholism, brain tumor, anxiety neurosis, hysteria, and psychosis.

Researchers have known for many years that psychological disturbances are one of the characteristic signs of nutritional deficiencies. A study titled *Disadvantaged Children* tells of severely ill youngsters who seemed to lose their natural curiosity. These cases, invariably, were those of severe protein-calorie malnutrition. The malnutrition of affluence does not necessarily cause protein-calorie deficiency, but it does bring on other problems that have just as striking an effect on behavior.

These behavioral studies, related to diet, ranged from observations on schizophrenia to alcoholism.

Dr. Josef Brozek, a prominent psychologist, is quoted in the book *Food Power: Nutrition and Your Child's Behavior* by Dr. Hugh Powers and James Presley, as saying: "Deficiency of all of the major nutrients, including water, eventually affects behavior even though the mechanisms involved will vary."

Dr. Ben Feingold in *Why Your Child Is Hyperactive* substantiates his claim that behavioral disturbances and learning disabilities often originate in the artificial food flavors and colors that are so much a part of junk food and food items not generally considered harmful.

Johnny one day deliberately ran his tricycle into the path of an oncoming car. At home he took out his frustrations in other ways—stomping, kicking walls during temper tantrums, surliness, telling big lies about little problems, and generally creating chaos.

A handsome boy, Johnny (not his real name) lived near San Francisco and started on his aberrant behavior kick at the age of five. His disposition was either up or down, seldom level. At school he couldn't concentrate, couldn't learn.

Johnny was blessed with strong, stable parents. A psychiatrist at a prominent medical center interviewed his parents and twelve-year-old brother, who was not similarly afflicted. The style of the family was one of quiet control. The psychiatrist concluded that everything was in order. "Goodness" was stressed, and the doctor wondered if perhaps Johnny was paying a high price for the family's commitment to "goodness."

But the mother was convinced that Johnny's difficulty stemmed from what he ate. Since crib days, the boy was restless and resisted cuddling. Long days of tests followed, but Johnny's behavioral problems continued.

Nearly six months of detailed reporting in a diary by his patient mother revealed that Johnny's behavior was triggered by certain added coloring found in unsuspected foods such as the barbecue sauce on potato chips, orange juice, candy, and other foods the average eater can ingest without difficulty.

After Johnny became attuned to a new diet, life became easier at home, at school, and within himself. The long search and careful recording of what he ate paid big dividends.

Alexander Schauss, director of the Institute for Biosocial Research, is convinced that criminals commit crimes not because they are born bad but because they *feel* bad. A criminal, he states in his book *Diet, Crime and Delinquency* doesn't break the law because his mother didn't love him. "He is bad because he *feels* bad," Dr. Schauss insists.

One murderer interviewed by the researcher was a young woman who had become paranoid due to an overactive thyroid gland. "In her hyperexcited state," he says, "she became fearful of her downstairs neighbor and killed her."

A young man was given the hormone testosterone by his doctor to treat impotence. The testosterone worked so well that the young man took several times the recommended doses. Consequently, this male sex hormone, which increases aggressiveness, drove him to high-pitched emotions. In such a state he had an argument with his girlfriend. In the heat of it he pulled out his pistol and "burned her."

Heroin addicts in Harlem were able to kick their habit faster when they first got off a diet of fast foods, colas, and refined sugar. Physical exercise was also an excellent treatment for relaxing the addicts' need for drugs. When they were able to throw off the dual sins of junk food and drugs, their appetites increased notably. Pale, thin junkies became healthy, happy, ruddy-faced men and women.

Barbara Reed, chief probation officer, Cuyahoga Falls Municipal Probation Department in Ohio, told the United States Senate Select Committee on Nutrition and Human Needs about her experiences with 318 offenders. Of these, she said, "Two hundred fifty-two required attention as to their diet and vitamin needs." Mrs. Reed added: "We have not had one single person back in court for trouble who has maintained and stayed on the nutritional diet."

One senator challenged her finding: "I wonder," he said, "how many of these success stories are because of diet and how many are because they may have been receiving special attention, someone cared about their rehabilitation."

Mrs. Reed replied, "I have been in this field for fourteen years. I was giving people a lot of loving attention before without nearly the results as now. The two work hand in hand . . . but, I just don't think kids on probation heard what we were talking about when they were so disconnected with reality that they couldn't remember what had been said. Now they do remember and it makes a big difference."

In conclusion, at the Senate hearing Mrs. Reed said: "Never before has the court had such a tool for working with the many ill people who find themselves in trouble. We wonder what the results would be if this method of treatment could also be applied to all those sentenced to jail."

The Reverend Benard Mason of Glendale, California, founder and director of the Hypoglycemia Research Fellowship of Southern California, is convinced that "junk food has given rise to all kinds of mental problems—problems which generate all kinds of behavior problems leading to senseless violent crimes."

Alcoholism, food allergies, and many excesses—how much of these among the 12 million arrests of children each year are the result of what is put into the stomach? The subject is worth all the attention we can give it—at home, at school, at work, and at play.

6

What a Parent Can Do

Sow a meal.
Cultivate a taste.
Sow a taste.
Reap a preference.
Sow a preference.
Reap a habit.
Sow a habit.
Reap health!

Good nutrition can be taught in creative ways to the delight of children. If correct habits have not been established early, the problem is more difficult but not overwhelming.

A child learns by example and experience what foods to eat. Dad is more influential than mother at mealtime. Mother is *supposed* to like the food, because she prepared it. If the child sees the father relishing his vegetables, the enthusiasm is contagious.

Variety is another key. A child who grows up eating

only a small variety of foods has a higher risk of being deficient in some food nutrients.

Parents need to refrain from passing on their prejudices. A woman who was forced to eat spinach when she was a child and learned to hate it, told this to a neighbor at lunch in front of her toddler. She gave a clear signal to the little boy that a certain food was undesirable.

The ages from birth to six years set the stage for a lifetime of eating preferences. Environment is important. If a child begins his years programmed to eat lean meats, fruits, vegetables, and an assortment of dairy products, he might not discover his sweet tooth until late in his childhood. Such a situation keeps health and figure intact.

Dr. George Owen and Mrs. Kathryn Kram of the Ohio State University Pediatrics Department have prepared a study on the eating habits of youngsters from one to six from all over the nation. The survey showed that 77 percent of those studied were willing to try new foods between the ages of one and two. By the time they were in the two-to-four category, their willingness dropped by 10 percent. In the year of their fourth anniversary their adventuresome spirit dropped by another 7 percent.

There is a direct link, the researchers found, between a child's lack of eating and his mother's degree of interest in preparing the food.

Social Research, Inc., an agency that has studied a thousand homemakers, concludes: Housewives are blissfully unaware of their families' nutritional needs. The sight of pale, anemic, listless youngsters or children tearing around trying desperately to outrun their sugar "crazies" is enough to make sad the hearts of those whose eyes have been opened to the bountiful blessings of wholesome food. What a legacy to leave a loved one!

An honest physician will admit: Medical schools teach a student doctor how to practice medicine. They offer one diet for diabetics . . . one diet for weight watchers . . . and one diet for heart patients. To the honest seekers for nutritional advice the doctors, in turn, offer a shrug. As for vitamin supplements: "They can't hurt you," or "It's your money, if you want to waste it."

To find out how to get children off junk food and into the nutrition scene, a homemaker is well advised to take a good look within her own kitchen. The trouble doesn't come from economy. Americans spend a hundred billion dollars every year for food. They are eating well but not wisely. Every year consumer habits grow worse. Half the American population, states the United States Department of Agriculture, do not eat a balanced diet. Substandard nutrition does not follow class, cultural, or economic lines.

Among the most neglected foods on American tables are: yellow and green vegetables, citrus fruits, and milk. The meal most often skipped is breakfast. Bodies are most likely to be deficient in vitamin A, vitamin C, calcium, and iron.

In days gone by, the dinner hour in the evening was a time for wrapping up the day together. Since one-third of all dinners now are eaten outside the home, this time for closely knit family fun and sharing is limited. Today dinner can be at any hour, sandwiched in between frenetic work and leisure.

A study of 3,500 high school students in Massachusetts showed that 11 percent of the boys and 19 percent of the girls ignored breakfast habitually. Those who did stop in the kitchen long enough to eat grabbed the first bit of fast food available and sped off to meet the day.

"At school," said Lendon Smith, a pediatrician speaking in La Canada, California, "we should ask the students which had breakfast. We should send home the ones who didn't because they don't have a brain anyhow."

Researchers at the University of Iowa discovered that

collegians who skipped breakfast required longer time to make decisions . . . were less steady . . . didn't produce as much work as the students who did stop to refuel.

"Small children," says Harvard University nutritionist Dr. Jean Mayer, "cannot last without a meal as long as adults because their metabolism is much faster. They burn things much more rapidly . . . so that small children cannot . . . function all morning if they have had no breakfast."

A survey of teen snack preferences showed that girls and boys put soft drinks, potato chips, pies, cakes, pastry, and cookies at the top.

"All advertising," Dr. Mayer lamented, "or just about all, is on the worthless foods. There is very little advertising for fruits and vegetables . . . advertising represents well over a billion dollars of expenditures, and it's all directed at the less useful foods. . . ."

A nutritional revolution has begun, turning our nation back to health. Won't you join, for the sake of the next generation?

Following are simple, innovative recipes that will serve as alternatives for jaded palates.

7

Breakfast

The first meal of the day is the most neglected, yet it is the most important. A good breakfast, using recipes like the following, will fortify a child's body and make him less hungry for junk food to keep going.

Simple whole fruits of the season served attractively are always welcomed. Whole fruit is preferable to fruit juice because of the additional fiber that is consumed. Most children lack adequate amounts of vitamin C, so don't overlook this vital area.

Consider a variety of choices for the child who doesn't like the usual eggs, cereal, and toast breakfast:

- Grilled cheese on whole wheat toast sandwich
- Pea soup made with milk
- Baked custard (sugarless) and protein-packed cookies
- Chipped beef on whole wheat toast
- Hot rice with raisins
- Cheese omelet
- High-protein breakfast drinks
- Bran muffins

Whatever your child enjoys that is rich in protein can make a good breakfast. Always include a glass of whole milk. Breakfast should meet at least one-fourth of the day's nutritional requirements.

Basic Bran Muffins

4 cups raw bran or bran buds
2 cups wheat germ (test for freshness)*
2 cups boiling water
1 cup corn oil
1½ cups honey
¼ cup blackstrap molasses
3 eggs
1 quart buttermilk
1½ cups enriched all-purpose flour
4 cups whole wheat flour
2 teaspoons salt
5 teaspoons baking soda
1 cup nuts or sesame seeds (optional)

Combine bran and wheat germ in 6-quart bowl. Stir in boiling water. Add oil, honey, molasses, eggs, and buttermilk.

Sift flours, salt, and baking soda together and blend into the liquid. Stir until all dry ingredients are just moistened. Fold in nuts or seeds. Fill muffin tins ⅔ full and bake in 350° F. oven for 12 to 14 minutes.

Makes 7 dozen muffins. Batter will keep in refrigerator for 4 weeks.

Variations

- Add grated orange rind, raisins, dates, chopped prunes, pineapple, or other fruit as desired.

* If wheat germ burns the throat when tasted, discard. It is rancid.

Blueberry Waffles

2 eggs, separated
1 cup nonfat liquid milk
1 tablespoon corn oil
¾ cup whole wheat flour
¼ cup cornmeal
⅓ cup raw bran flakes
¼ teaspoon salt
1 teaspoon baking powder
1 cup drained blueberries

Separate eggs, beat whites until stiff. Add milk and oil to yolks and blend. Stir in dry ingredients and beat until smooth. Fold in whites. Spoon onto hot waffle griddle. Bake until steaming stops. Serve immediately.

Makes 2 waffles; recipe easily doubled.

Breakfast Shake

1 cup milk
1 cup plain yogurt
1 ripe banana
2 tablespoons fresh wheat germ
3 tablespoons honey or molasses
4 ice cubes

Combine all ingredients in blender. Whirl for 2 minutes.

Serves 2.

Variations

- Add ½ cup fresh or frozen strawberries or blueberries.
- Add pitted prunes or dates.
- Add ½ cup peach or apricot slices.

Strawberry Smoothie

1 cup strawberries, fresh or frozen
1 cup nonfat liquid milk
6 frozen cubes of buttermilk*
1 tablespoon fructose granules or honey
1 egg

Combine all ingredients in blender and whirl until smooth and thick. Serve immediately.

Variations

- Use unsweetened pineapple juice if allergic to milk.
- Add 1 tablespoon brewer's yeast.
- Add 2 tablespoons protein powder.

* Pour buttermilk into ice cube tray and freeze several hours. Keep plenty on hand for all blender drinks.

English-French Toast

4 eggs
1 cup milk
¼ teaspoon salt
dash of pepper and nutmeg
4 English muffins

Beat eggs; add milk and seasonings. Pour in shallow dish. Dip 8 muffin halves on both sides and let stand to absorb all liquid. Place on lightly oiled hot griddle and brown on both sides.

Serve with fresh sliced strawberries or orange marmalade or both. Top with spoonful of sour cream.

Serves 4.

Oatmeal Raisin Muffins
(wheat free)

1 cup rolled oats
1 cup buttermilk
½ cup oil (polyunsaturated)
⅓ cup honey or molasses
1 egg well beaten
1 cup plus 2 tablespoons oat flour
½ teaspoon salt
½ teaspoon soda
1½ teaspoons baking powder
⅓ cup moist raisins

Mix oats and buttermilk together and let stand at least 30 minutes.

Stir together oil, honey, and egg and add to oatmeal mixture, blending well.

Add dry ingredients and mix just until all is moistened. Fold in raisins.

Spoon into foil-lined muffin tins. Bake in 350° F. oven for 25 minutes.

Makes 1 dozen.

Our Favorite Granola

7 cups rolled oats, uncooked
1 cup sunflower seeds, crushed in blender
½ cup sesame seeds, crushed in blender
1 cup almonds—or pecans, cashews, peanuts, or walnuts (crush in plastic bag with rolling pin)
1 cup unprocessed bran flakes (eliminate bran if allergic to wheat)
¼ cup soy granules (lecithin)
1 teaspoon iodized salt
1 cup soy oil
1 cup pure honey
1 tablespoon vanilla

Bake oats in large baking pan with enough room to stir, (18″ × 12″) for 10 minutes in preheated 325° F. oven.

Remove pan from oven and add seeds, nuts, bran, lecithin, and salt. Mix well. Pour oil, honey, and vanilla over dry ingredients and stir until blended. Return to oven and reduce heat to 300°. Bake for another 25 to 30 minutes, stirring often to keep oats from scorching. Cool. Crumble and store in airtight container.

At serving time sprinkle with:

- wheat germ (keep in refrigerator because it can become rancid)
- moist raisins or chopped prunes
- chopped apple or sliced banana

Silver Dollar Griddle Cakes

3 eggs, beaten
½ cup low-fat cottage cheese
½ cup nonfat liquid milk
2 tablespoons margarine, melted
1 cup whole wheat flour
⅛ teaspoon salt
½ teaspoon baking powder

Blend eggs, cottage cheese, margarine, and milk in blender until smooth.

Sift flour, salt, and baking powder into mixing bowl. Pour liquid over flour and mix thoroughly.

Bake batter the size of silver dollars on a hot griddle, lightly oiled.

Serve with apple butter, apricot butter, or warm honey heated with butter.

Lumberjack Apple Cookies

1 stick margarine or butter
¾ cup honey
1 egg
1⅓ cups whole wheat flour
1 teaspoon soda
⅛ teaspoon baking powder
½ teaspoon cinnamon
¼ teaspoon cloves
¼ teaspoon allspice
2 teaspoons vanilla
1½ cups oats
1½ cups raw apple, grated
½ cup moist raisins

Beat margarine and honey until smooth. Add egg and blend well.

Measure flour, soda, baking powder, and spices into sifter. Sift into honey mixture in small amounts and stir thoroughly. Add vanilla and oats and blend. Fold in grated apple and raisins.

Drop cookie dough by teaspoon onto lightly oiled cookie sheet. Bake for 15 minutes in 350° F. oven.

Makes 45 to 50 2″ cookies.

8

Lunch

Brown bag, thermos, or gourmet meal, lunch gives youngsters go power for an active afternoon. Use these recipes, and creative ones of your own, to make this second half of the day brighter for the pint-sized eaters who look to you for their very lives.

Brown Bag Lunch Ideas

A nutritious lunch should include:

- A protein-rich food such as fish, poultry, meat, cheese, eggs, or nut butter
- Crisp finger food such as broccoli buds, cauliflower, cucumbers, carrots, celery, green pepper, jicama, or radishes (pickles can be an extra treat if desired)
- Fresh fruit
- A serving of nuts, sugarless cookies, sugarless cupcake, or nut breads

- Generous serving of milk (if allergic to milk use cans of pure fruit juices, not juice drinks or pop)

Suggestions for the lunch menu:

- Meat loaf on whole wheat bread
- Sardines on whole-grain crackers
- Baked crunchy chicken with a carton of potato salad
- Peanut butter whipped with powdered milk, orange juice, and chopped dates and spread on oatmeal or whole wheat bread
- Turkey sliced thin or chopped with mayonnaise and spread on rye bread (add alfalfa sprouts)
- Deviled ham mixed with thawed frozen peas and a little mayonnaise
- Chicken livers pureed and mixed with celery, mayonnaise, and minced onion.

Cabbage Melt

1 cup finely chopped cabbage
1 tablespoon sour cream
1 tablespoon mayonnaise
1 tablespoon catsup
2 tablespoons green pepper finely diced
3 green onions, finely diced
8 sourdough English Muffins
1 cup shredded cheddar or Monterey Jack cheese

Mix cream, mayonnaise, catsup, pepper, and onions together. Combine this dressing mixture with the cabbage. Spread onto 8 sourdough English-muffin halves. Cover generously with cheese. Place under broiler until cheese melts. If you prefer, mixture can be spread onto whole wheat bread slices, or French sourdough.

Silly Salad

For each individual salad:

1 cup fresh alfalfa sprouts
½ cup shredded carrots
2 tablespoons shredded coconut
2 tablespoons sliced celery
1 tablespoon crushed peanuts or cashews

Place alfalfa sprouts on salad plate evenly; sprinkle with carrots, then coconut, then celery, and top with nuts. Pour lemon-lime dressing, or child's favorite, over top.

Note: You may prefer to toss the ingredients with the dressing. Do what appeals to your child and help the youngster to enjoy salads at an early age.

Hobo Bread

1⅓ cups raisins or currants
2 teaspoons baking soda
1 cup boiling water
½ cup molasses
½ stick margarine
1 egg
2 cups whole wheat flour
¼ teaspoon salt
¼ cup chopped nuts

Sprinkle soda over raisins. Pour water over raisins and soda. Cool.

Beat together molasses, margarine, and egg. Sift flour with salt. Add slowly to molasses mixture. Blend well. Add nuts.

With a piece of wax paper grease two one-pound coffee cans generously. Sprinkle a little flour into the can and roll can so flour covers bottom and all sides.

Divide mixture between cans. Bake in 350° F. oven for one hour. Remove cans using large pot holders so you won't get burned. Place upside down on wire rack and cool. Serve while still warm. Keeps well, wrapped in foil.

Pocket Full of Energy

Pita Bread, or Pocket Bread, Sandwich

Fillings to choose from: (use a protein and several fresh vegetables)

coleslaw
tuna
chopped tomatoes
lettuce
anchovies
sardines
alfalfa sprouts
grated cheese
minced green onions
minced green bell pepper
olives

Quick Pizza Treat

2 tablespoons olive oil
4 green onions, finely diced
1 cup pizza sauce
½ teaspoon Italian seasoning
½ fresh green or red bell pepper, diced
1 small jar green olives, sliced
¼ cup sliced black olives
½ cup fresh sliced mushrooms
1 pound sharp cheddar cheese, shredded

Heat oil and saute onions for three minutes.

Blend all the ingredients together in a mixing bowl. Spread on sourdough bread and broil until cheese is bubbly. English muffins or large crackers can be used instead of bread.

This will keep for several days in the refrigerator. Great to have on hand for after-school snacks.

Party Sandwiches

12 French rolls
¾ pound grated cheddar cheese
1 pint pitted ripe olives, chopped
3 fresh green onions, chopped
1 green pepper, chopped
4 hard-cooked eggs, chopped
1 medium tomato, diced
⅛ teaspoon salt
dash of cayenne pepper
4 tablespoons cider vinegar
8-ounce can tomato sauce

Cut tops off rolls, scoop out centers (reserve for crumbs), and butter inside.

Mix all the remaining ingredients together, adding the vinegar and tomato sauce last. Mixture should be thick. Add the sauce slowly to determine if all is needed. Fill rolls generously. Replace top, wrap in wax paper, and twist ends closed.

Bake in 350° F. oven on cookie sheet for about 30 minutes. Allow to set 15 minutes before serving.

Serves 6 to 12 hearty appetites.

Sandwiches can be made in advance and frozen. Allow some thawing time before baking.

Vege-Taco

3 tablespoons butter
1 bunch green onions, diced
4 small zucchini squash, thinly sliced (after brushing clean, taste to see if skin is mild—if bitter, peel off skin)
½ green bell pepper, minced
1 cup fresh mushrooms, diced
¼ cup cashews or walnuts, crushed
1 ripe avocado, diced
2 cups natural cheddar cheese, grated
alfalfa sprouts
1 dozen tortillas

Melt butter and sauté vegetables together for 5 to 7 minutes. Stir in nuts. Place in bowl.

Fry tortilla quickly in hot corn oil. Blot on paper towel. Place helping of hot vegetables onto tortilla followed by cheese, avocado, and alfalfa sprouts. Fold over and enjoy.

9

Dinner

For the best of health,
eat breakfast like a king,
lunch like a prince, and
dinner like a pauper.

Following are suggested recipes for replacing the processed foods so readily available. Getting your kids off junk food will be worth the effort put into preparing these recipes.

Baked Chicken a la Parsley

1 cup evaporated milk
1 bunch parsley, dipped in salted water and rinsed
1 large onion, finely chopped
½ stick butter or margarine, melted
1 teaspoon poultry seasoning
1 teaspoon black or white pepper
2 cups crushed cornflakes
1 frying chicken

Pour milk into a 9″ × 13″ baking pan and cover with parsley and onion.

Melt butter and add poultry seasoning and pepper and blend. Dip chicken in butter and then roll in finely crushed cornflakes. Place chicken on top of parsley and sprinkle with paprika. Bake in 350° F. oven for 15 minutes. Reduce heat to 325° and bake for 1 hour and 15 minutes.

Baked Potato Sticks

4 smooth medium-sized potatoes
2 slightly beaten egg whites
parmesan cheese
sesame seeds or poppy seeds

Scrub potatoes with a stiff brush and trim if necessary. Cut each potato into 8 to 10 sticks. Brush with the egg white and sprinkle each stick generously with the parmesan cheese (some sticks can be sprinkled with sesame seeds or poppy seeds). Place sticks on a cookie sheet and bake for 30 to 35 minutes in a preheated 425° F. oven. Serve immediately.

Serves 6 to 8.

Variations:

- Sprinkle with minced parsley or dill weed.
- Cover with foil for part of the baking time for a softer stick.

Carrot-Peanut Loaf

1 egg
¼ cup nonfat dry milk
½ cup pure peanut butter, thinned with 2 tablespoons)liquid milk
1½ cups finely grated carrots
1 cup cooked brown rice
¼ cup ground sunflower seeds
1 tablespoon orange juice
1 cup ground peanuts (blender is fine for this)

Beat egg, powdered milk, and peanut butter. Stir in the remaining ingredients and blend. Fill buttered 9¼″ × 5¼″ × 3″ loaf pan and bake in 325° F. oven for 1 hour or until nicely browned.

Bean Burgers

2 cups cooked, mashed beans (pinto, kidney, garbanzos, or Great Northern)
2 green onions, thinly sliced
1 tablespoon margarine or butter
2 tablespoons fresh minced parsley
6 crackers (Ry-krisp type) rolled fine
cheese

In large skillet sauté green onions in butter. Add beans, parsley, and crackers. Mix together well. Form into 4 patties.

In another skillet heat 1 tablespoon corn oil and brown patties over moderate heat for about 4 minutes on each side.

Serves 4.

Optional: Top with strips of cheese and place under broiler until cheese is melted.

Chicken Delight Salad

1 cup cooked brown rice

Marinade:
¼ cup vegetable oil
2 tablespoons lemon juice
1 tablespoon honey or other sweetener
1 teaspoon paprika
1 teaspoon salt
1 green bell pepper, chopped
2 tablespoons minced chives

* * *

5 cups cooked, diced chicken
2½ cups diced celery

Dressing:
½ cup sour cream
1 tablespoon cream or milk
½ cup mayonnaise
2 tablespoons soy sauce
dash of ginger

Toss rice with the marinade. Allow to stand in refrigerator while preparing chicken and dressing.

Place chicken in chilled bowl, add rice, celery and dressing. Toss again.

Serve on crisp lettuce leaf garnished with crab apples, fresh grapes, or cantaloupes in season.

Curried Chicken for Two

2 chicken breasts, boned and cut into strips (reserve bones)
lemon
1 tablespoon peanut oil
1 tablespoon margarine
3 to 4 teaspoons curry powder
1 cup chicken broth
salt and pepper to taste
3 teaspoons cornstarch
3 tablespoons water
coconut

One hour beforehand squeeze fresh lemon over chicken and chill.

Place bones in 1½ cups seasoned water and cook for 60 minutes.

When broth is ready, heat margarine and oil in skillet, add curry powder, and cook 3 minutes. Add chicken, stirring to blend into sauce. Pour broth over chicken and cover skillet. Simmer gently 10 minutes.

Mix cornstarch with water and add to chicken. Cook 2 minutes until liquid is slightly thickened and clear.

Sprinkle with coconut, garnish with pineapple, papaya, or fruits in season, and serve with hot rice.

Serves 2.

Vegetable Soup

1½ cups Great Northern dried beans, sorted, rinsed
1 quart tomato juice
1 large bay leaf
2 onions, chopped
2 cloves fresh garlic, minced
2 teaspoons salt
1 teaspoon pepper
1 cup celery, chopped
1 large potato, peeled and chopped
8 carrots, peeled and sliced
4 turnips, peeled and chopped
1 10-ounce package frozen corn
¼ cup chopped parsley

Cover beans with water and soak overnight in 6-quart kettle.

Place kettle of beans, undrained, on high heat and bring to a boil. Skim off foam. Add 1 quart water, tomato juice, bay leaf, onions, garlic, salt, and pepper. Cover and simmer 2½ hours. Add all the vegetables and simmer 1 hour longer. Adjust seasoning.

Serves 12. Freeze leftovers.

Mushroom Stroganoff

2 tablespoons butter
1 medium onion, finely chopped
1 clove garlic, grated fine
3 tablespoons fresh parsley, minced
2 to 3 cups fresh mushrooms, halved or quartered, depending on size
1 cup cottage cheese
½ cup powdered milk
½ cup plain yogurt
1 egg, slightly beaten

In saucepan melt butter and add the onion and garlic. Sauté until clear but not brown. Add parsley and mushrooms and cook over low heat about 5 minutes, stirring often.

Mix cheese, milk, yogurt, and egg together. Add to vegetables and keep on heat just long enough to heat through. Sprinkle with salt and pepper.

Serve hot over steaming brown rice or hot buttered spinach noodles.

Carrot Meat Loaf

½ cup nonfat liquid milk
1 egg, beaten
1 cup bread cubes or dressing mix
½ onion, chopped
1 tablespoon soy sauce
1 teaspoon salt
¼ teaspoon pepper
1 pound lean ground beef
1 cup grated carrots
½ cup chopped bean sprouts
¼ cup finely diced celery

Place milk, egg, bread, onion, soy sauce, pepper, and salt in blender. Whirl.

Place lean ground beef in large mixing bowl with carrots, sprouts, and celery. Pour liquid over meat and mix well with hands. Pat into a 9″ × 5″ × 3″ loaf pan or 8″ × 8″ × 2″ pan or bake this mixture in a 12-cup muffin tin. Fill cups to the top and bake in half the time. You'll have a small amount left over from a 12-cup tin, so make a tiny loaf and bake in a small pie plate at the same time. Bake for one hour in 350° F. oven.

(Our sons like a couple of meat muffins in their school lunches.)

Carob Pudding
(no eggs)

½ cup carob powder (unsweetened)
3 tablespoons cornstarch
⅓ cup fructose granules
⅛ teaspoon salt
1 cup nonfat liquid milk
1 cup whipping cream, whipped until it holds a peak
1 teaspoon vanilla
1 teaspoon maple flavoring

Combine carob, cornstarch, fructose, and salt in double boiler. Stir, adding milk, until smooth. Cook over simmering water and stir until thickened. Add vanilla and maple flavoring. Cool well. Fold in whipped cream and spoon into sherbet dishes or parfait glasses. Sliced bananas are a delicious addition.

Carrot Yogurt Cake

2 eggs or 4 egg whites
½ stick margarine or butter
¼ cup molasses
¼ cup honey or fructose
1 cup plain yogurt
½ cup apple juice
2 cups whole wheat flour
⅓ cup fresh wheat germ
½ teaspoon nutmeg
1½ teaspoons cinnamon
1½ teaspoons baking soda
1 cup finely grated carrots (raw or cooked)

Beat eggs and margarine together in large mixing bowl. Add molasses, honey, yogurt, and juice. Blend well.

Measure dry ingredients and lightly mix together.

Add to egg mixture and combine thoroughly. Fold in grated carrots. Pour into 9″ × 13″ cake pan coated with nonstick spray. Bake at 325° for about 1 hour. Test center with toothpick.

Instant Cherry Tortes

12 graham crackers
1 cup skim ricotta cheese or cottage cheese
2 tablespoons honey or 2 tablespoons fructose granules
½ teaspoon vanilla
1½ cups cherries, fresh or canned
¾ cup whipped cream
1 tablespoon honey
½ teaspoon vanilla
½ cup crushed nuts

There will be 4 stacks of graham crackers, with 3 crackers to a stack, with filling in between.

Mix cheese, honey, and vanilla together.

Beat whipped cream until thick, and add honey and vanilla.

For one torte:

Spread about one tablespoon of cheese mixture onto each of 3 graham crackers. Place 9 cherries on top of one cracker. Top with a graham cracker spread with cheese. Add 9 cherries on top. Place 3rd graham cracker on top of cherries.

Frost each stack with whipped cream mixture. Sprinkle with finely crushed nuts. Place in refrigerator and chill for several hours.

Makes 4 tortes.

Maple Pecan White Fudge

⅓ cup butter, softened
½ cup pure maple syrup
1¼ cups powdered milk* (noninstant, available at health food stores)
⅓ cup coarsely chopped pecans

Beat together butter and maple syrup. Add dry milk in small amounts and beat until smooth. Mixture should be heavy. Add nuts and press into 8″ × 8″ pan coated with nonstick spray. Chill well before cutting.

* If using instant powdered milk you will need more. Add enough to have a thick consistency.

Molasses Flan

2 tablespoons molasses
3¼ cups evaporated skimmed milk (2 13-ounce cans)
¼ cup water
2-inch sliver of lemon rind
stick cinnamon
2 whole eggs
3 egg whites
3 tablespoons fructose
⅛ teaspoon salt
1 tablespoon vanilla

Coat sides of a 4 to 6-cup ring mold with molasses.

Scald milk and water for 5 to 7 minutes with lemon rind and cinnamon stick. Avoid boiling.

Beat eggs with fructose and salt.

Remove lemon rind and cinnamon stick from milk and blend milk mixture into eggs. Add vanilla. Strain carefully into mold and set in pan containing 1 inch of hot water. Bake in 325° F. oven for about 50 minutes or until set. Remove mold immediately from pan and cool on rack. Chill several hours.

At serving time, carefully loosen edges of custard with a sharp knife. Cover mold with a chilled serving plate and invert. Allow molasses syrup to drain over flan and then remove mold.

Serves 6.

Papa's Prune Whip

2 cups prunes
¾ cup orange juice
1 cup whipping cream
½ teaspoon cinnamon
1 teaspoon vanilla

Place prunes in small saucepan. Add orange juice and cook slowly for 10 minutes. Cool. Remove pits from prunes and chop prunes (on plastic cutting board if you have one). Place prunes in refrigerator to chill.

Beat whipping cream until thick. Add vanilla and cinnamon and fold in the cold prunes. Pour into sherbet or parfait glasses. Custard cups can also be used. Sprinkle top with a litttle nutmeg and place glasses in refrigerator until serving time.

Serves 6.

Rice Pudding
(no eggs or cow's milk)

2 cups cooked rice (brown preferably)
¼ cup honey, molasses, or fructose granules
1 cup raisins or chopped dates
1 cup grated apple or crushed pineapple (unsweetened and well drained)
1 cup soy milk

Combine ingredients and pour into 2-quart baking dish. Place dish in a shallow pan. Pour hot water into pan to about 1 inch. Bake in 350° F. oven for 30 minutes or until mixture is set.

Serves 8.

Rusty's Fig Newts

Cookie Dough
1½ cups sifted whole wheat flour
1½ cups sifted enriched all-purpose flour
4 teaspoons cream of tartar
2 teaspoons soda
1 teaspoon salt
2 tablespoons fructose
2 tablespoons lecithin granules
2 tablespoons safflower or corn oil
2 egg whites
1 stick margarine, softened
1 tablespoon lemon juice
¼ cup water

Sift dry ingredients together into large mixing bowl. Stir in oil, egg whites, margarine, and lemon juice. Add water, stirring with wooden spoon until mixture holds together. Form into a ball, cover, and chill one hour.

Filling
1 pound dried figs, finely chopped (2 cups)
½ cup water
½ cup fresh orange juice, unsweetened

Combine ingredients in blender and whirl. Pour into saucepan and gently simmer for 10 minutes. Cool.

Roll half of the dough to ⅛″ thickness on floured board into a rectangle about 8″ × 14″ long. Cut lengthwise so there are two strips 4″ × 14″. Spread filling in center of each strip and fold dough over from each side and seal. Cut into about 1¾″ bars. Place bars seam side down on oiled cookie sheet. Bake in 350° oven for 15 minutes.

Makes approximately 44.

Strawberry Yogurt Mousse

2 envelopes unflavored gelatin
½ cup fructose granules
⅛ teaspoon salt
3 eggs, separated
1 cup nonfat liquid milk
2 cups strawberry yogurt (no sugar)
1 cup whipping cream

Combine gelatin, ¼ cup fructose, and salt in saucepan.

Beat together egg yolks and milk in bowl and stir into gelatin mixture. Cook over low heat, stirring constantly to dissolve gelatin, about 5 minutes. Cool, and blend in yogurt. Chill well.

Beat egg whites, gradually adding ¼ cup fructose until mixture is thick and holds a peak.

Whip cream until thickened and fold into egg whites. Add to strawberry mixture, folding to blend well.

This can be spooned into parfait or sherbet glasses and garnished with fresh fruit. Or, the mixture can be turned into an 8-cup mold and chilled for several hours before unmolding. Serve on bed of lettuce or trim with mint leaves.

Virginia's Mud Balls
(Carob Treat)

1½ cups quick oats or old-fashioned rolled oats
¼ cup crushed sunflower seeds or chopped nuts
½ cup powdered nonfat milk
½ stick margarine or butter
½ cup honey
¼ cup carob powder, unsweetened
1 teaspoon vanilla
½ cup crunchy or smooth pure peanut butter
additional dry milk for finishing touch

Stir together oats, seeds, and dry milk.

Slowly melt margarine in saucepan; add honey and carob, blending well. Bring to a boil, stirring constantly, and boil for one minute. Remove from heat and beat in vanilla and peanut butter. Pour over oat mixture. Mix well. Form into walnut-sized balls, and roll in powdered milk or finely crushed peanuts. Store covered in refrigerator. They taste better the second day.

Makes about 34 to 36.

10

A Gift of Love

While strolling through the famous Huntington Art Gallery of Pasadena, California, we were smitten by the beauty of oil paintings dating to the eighteenth and nineteenth centuries. *Blue Boy* by Gainsborough, *Pinkie* by Sir Thomas Lawrence, *Lady with a Plume* by Rembrandt, and many other paintings silently attested to the skill of the artists.

How magnificent it would be, we thought, *to leave behind a legacy like that! What are we giving to succeeding generations as a result of our short pilgrimage?*

Then it struck us. Involved as we are with natural food, we realized that we are orchestrating the kitchen to create enduring health in our children. With the spatula as our brush and the breadboard as our palette, we are painting cheeks pink, putting sparkle into eyes and strength into bones, teeth, and muscle. The image of our children might never hang on a museum's wall or be printed in a collection of art, but they would give to their children and to their children's children a heritage that money cannot buy: glowing health.

Join us by leaving to your family this gift of love. Whether you are young or old, male or female, consider adopting the following resolutions and letting them be your special legacy:

1. Establish early a reverence for food as a beautiful gift from a loving Creator.
2. Expose children to a great variety of wholesome food. Let them experience and enjoy all types of flavors and textures of food.
3. Let them see mother and dad relish natural food. Fathers have more influence upon a child's taste preference than mothers. Encourage adults to be mature and to keep quiet about their own prejudices. Discourage criticism of wholesome food.
4. Do not give food as a reward or withhold it as punishment. Rather, accept it each day as a sacred gift necessary for good health.
5. Spend quality time in the kitchen and teach that cooking is a loving art not a drudgery. Emphasize both the beauty in food and their ultimate source of health and vitality.
6. If a person has genuinely tried to enjoy a food, but the body seems to reject it, accept that as valid—at least for the time being.
7. Major on natural and raw foods and minor on the synthetic, artificial, and factory-processed food.
8. Refrain from purchasing food that is of no nutritional value.
9. Consider the use of supplemental vitamins to assure adequate supplies of nutrients for maximum health.
10. Study the charts in the appendix as a guide to providing supplements for children and adults.

There may be answers in this book to questions you have never asked. We hope that your consciousness has been raised, that you will find the will to practice what we've suggested, and that your rewards will be abundant.

Eat right and feel great. It's the answer.

Appendix A

Vitamins with Iron for Children

A (acetate—water-dispersible)	5,000 I.U.
D (cholecalciferol)	400 I.U.
C (ascorbic acid and sodium ascorbate) . . .	75 mg.
B_1 (thiamine mononitrate)	2 mg.
B_2 (riboflavin)	2 mg.
B_6 (pyridoxine hydrochloride)	2 mg.
B_{12} (cobalamin concentrate)	5 mcg.
Folic Acid	200 mcg.
Pantothenic Acid (D-panthenol)	5 mg.
Biotin	150 mcg.
Niacinamide	20 mg.
E (as DL-AlphaTocopheryl acetate)	15 I.U.
Iron (ferrous fumarate)	10 mg.

Suggested Dosage: One tablet daily or as directed by doctor.

Source: Recommended for good health by the National Research Council

When buying a formula similar to this, look for a product that contains no artificial colors, artificial flavors, artificial sweeteners, or sucrose.

Appendix B

Fortified Vitamin and Mineral Insurance Formula

A daily dosage of six tablets provides:

A (palmitate)	15,000 I.U.
D (cholecalciferol)	400 I.U.
E (alpha tocopherol)	400 I.U.
K (phylloquinone)	100 mcg.
C (ascorbic acid)	2,500 mg.
B_1 (thiamine mononitrate)	20 mg.
B_2 (riboflavin)	20 mg.
B_3 (niacinamide)	200 mg.
B_6 (pyridoxine hydrochloride)	30 mg.
B_{12} (cobalamin concentrate)	90 mcg.
Pantothenic Acid	150 mg.
Biotin	3,000 mcg.
Folic Acid	400 mcg.
Choline	500 mg.
Inositol	500 mg.
Rutin	200 mg.
Para-aminobenzoic Acid	30 mg.
Calcium	250 mg.
Phosphorus	250 mg.
Magnesium	200 mg.
Iron (ferrous fumarate)	30 mg.

Zinc	30 mg.
Copper	2 mg.
Iodine	0.15 mg.
Manganese	10 mg.
Molybdenum	200 mcg.
Chromium (yeast)	200 mcg.
Selenium (yeast)	100 mcg.

Source: This specially formulated high potency multivitamin and mineral supplement was designed by Dr. Roger J. Williams of the Clayton Foundation Biochemical Institute, University of Texas, Austin. It provides the completeness of all the vitamins and minerals in the original Insurance Formula in higher amounts. It is manufactured by Bronson Pharmaceuticals, a direct-mail-order firm.